# BREW YOUR MEDICINE

## How To Use Basic Kitchen Equipment to Brew Custom Herbal Beer

Kristi Shapla

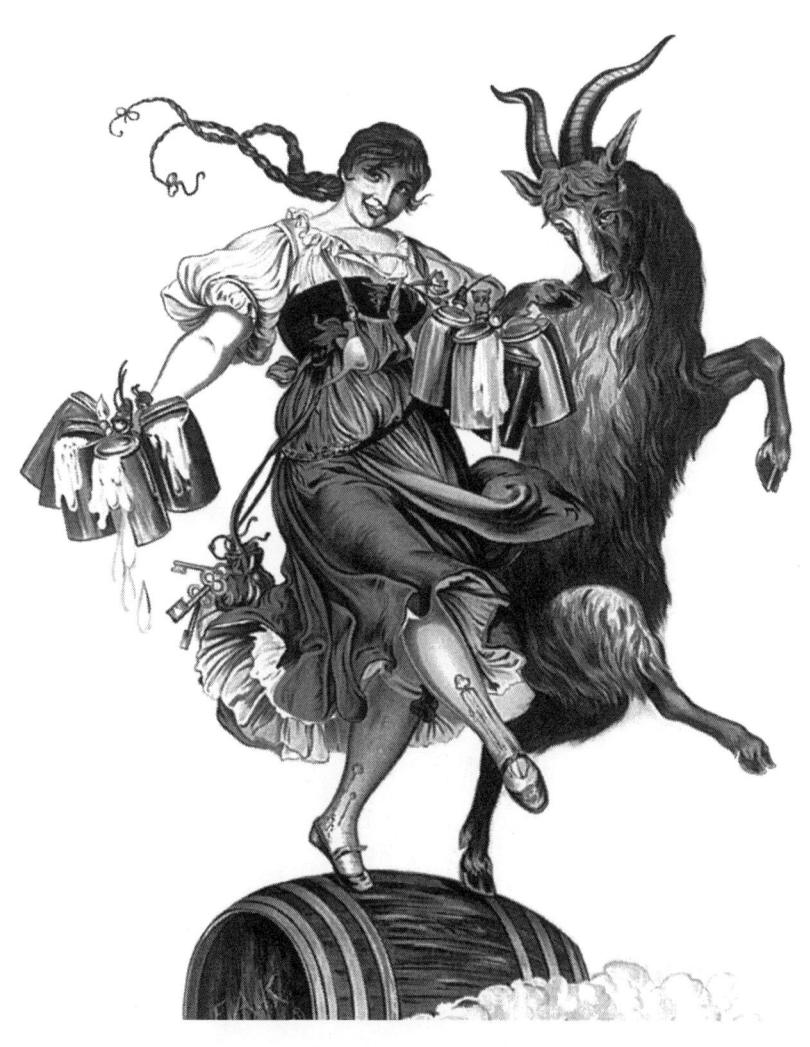

Copyright © 2012 Kristi Shapla

All rights reserved.

ISBN: 1475183127
ISBN-13: 978-1475183122

# CONTENTS

Introduction..................................................................i

Why Herbal Beer?........................................................1

A Simple Homebrew Setup......................................4

Ingredients..................................................................9

Keeping It Clean......................................................15

Brewing Stages.........................................................18

Instructions for 3 Types of Brewing....................24

Custom Herbal Formulas......................................31

Recipes (Beer).........................................................37

Save the Dregs! (Cooking Recipes)....................51

Appendix A: Roasting Roots & Grains...............57

Appendix B: Herb & Brewing Resources..........58

Bibliography & Further Reading.........................60

Index..........................................................................62

# INTRODUCTION

This book is written for anyone who enjoys beer, using herbs in their daily lives, or just wants to delve into an entirely new (but actually ancient) form of medicine making. All you need is a couple of large pots, some jugs, and a DIY spirit! You can easily craft your own medicinal beers to help tonify you through the seasons, aid in digestion, relax, and treat a myriad of discomforts.

My recipes are simple and straightforward. Most self-respecting beer making snobs might scoff at this simplicity. But my goal is not to make the perfect lager; it is to make an irresistibly tasty medicinal brew that is easy enough for anyone to make without the specialized, expensive equipment necessary for making those complex beers. Although, each time I give a beer snob a sample of my medicinal brew, I always get a fascinated thumbs up.

Whether you decide to continue crafting small batches of beer for yourself, or decide to make the jump to larger batches and more equipment, this book gives you a solid brewing foundation. I offer three variations of basic beer techniques, and then focus on good herbal formulating for tasty, healing brews.

One of the most important qualities of a good brewer is confidence! Just know that this is a very simple, foolproof process that has been carried out for millennia. Your brew will be the best you've ever tasted!

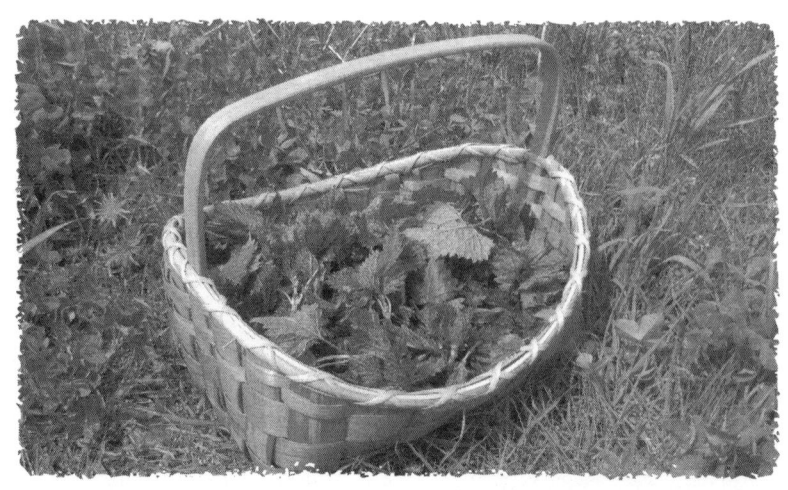

## WHY HERBAL BEER?

The use of herbs in beer and other fermented beverages goes back several millennia. In China, scientists believe fermented herbal beverages were being brewed 9,000 years ago! They have found hawthorne, jujube, sweet clover, jasmine, and hemp residues on brewing vessels made of clay. In Egypt, archaeologists have uncovered medical prescriptions written on papyrus from 1600 B.C. which included herbal beers as therapy. They were using tree resins such as frankincense, myrrh, pine, and fir, along with herbs such as coriander, cumin, mandrake, and wormwood.

These brews provided much needed nutrition for the intense, hard labor of that time, and everyone drank them, even children. Of course, the alcohol content of early brews was often much lower than modern beer, because the focus was not always inebriation.  Early beers served as a safe means of hydration, when water itself was often tainted with harmful bacteria.  Beer was also an effective sedative, analgesic, and disinfectant.  It's mind altering effects were used in religious and funerary ceremonies.  Herbs helped to highlight any of these aspects the brewer desired.

For us modern brewers, beer can be our medicine, and our daily vitamin supplement.  Since herbal therapies work best when taken on a consistent basis, I believe the easiest way to take herbs is in a form that we are already accustomed to: beer!

From an herbal perspective, herbal beer is an excellent way to preserve and magnify the benefits of seasonal herbs.  Dried herbs work wonderfully, too.  For the practitioner, client compliance is always a concern.  Most clients would happily drink a beer a day.  I find it is a very empowering skill to learn and teach.

Also, herbal beers can be made and ready to drink in as little as two weeks.  Not so great for acute conditions, but perfect for chronic conditions.  Herbal wines and meads are also a great low-alcohol preparation (and they are the first ferments I ever made), but they can take up to a year before they are drinkable when brewed at medicinal strength.  I find that with beer, I am able to concentrate the amount of herbs I use much higher and still have a great tasting beverage.

Fermentation activates and magnifies all of the active compounds, vitamins, and minerals that are present in herbs. These compounds are made bio-available by the yeast, so that they are readily absorbed by the body when consumed. Also, the yeast manufacture a whole host of their own vitamins in the process, including the all-important B vitamins. So, perhaps the real question is, Why NOT Herbal Beers?

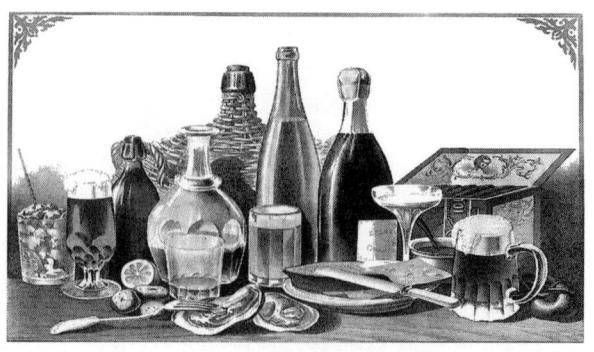

# A SIMPLE HOMEBREW SETUP

I hope this book will make it possible to brew your own herbal beers with very little in the way of investing in specialized equipment. Though, you just might catch the homebrewing bug and want those items. In which case, I suggest you look up some of the books and web sites I review in the back of this book for more in-depth details about the brewing process. So in this section, I'll discuss the bare minimum of tools and equipment necessary to get your first batch brewing.

For all equipment, I prefer to use stainless steel or glass. It is easier to sterilize, and won't react when decocting the herbs.

**Basic Kitchenware**:

Measuring cups

Scale

Large Sieve

    Or strainer lined with cloth

2 Pots large enough to hold 1.5 gallons each

    (to strain back and forth in)

Large stirring spoons

Thermometer

2, 1 Gallon Jugs

    (apple juice jugs work great)

**Other Essentials:**

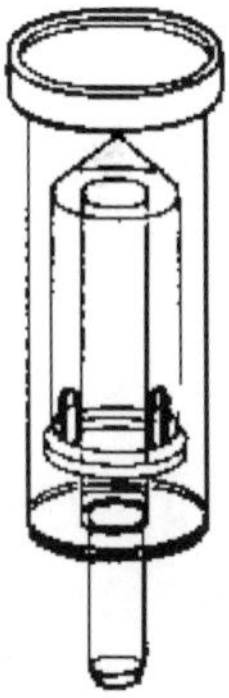

Some type of airlock is needed to allow gas to escape and keep insects, etc out. My favorite kind is pictured here. They are much easier to clean than the kind with chambers. This fits into a rubber stopper that fits perfectly into the apple juice jug. Stoppers come in all different sizes. Unfortunately, so do gallon jug mouths. I have acquired a variety of sizes over the years. You might try measuring the opening on your jug. Below is the size chart for rubber stoppers. Match the diameter of the mouth of your jug to the "Average Diameter" column below for the correct size.

| Stopper Size | Average Diameter |
|:---:|:---:|
| #2 | 11/16" |
| #3 | 13/16" |
| #5.5 | 1" |
| #6 | 1 1/8" |
| #6.5 | 1 1/4" |
| #7 | 1 5/16" |
| #7.5 | 1 3/8" |
| #8 | 1 7/16" |
| #8.5 | 1 9/16" |
| #9.5 | 1 5/8" |
| #10 | 1 13/16" |

Alternatively, you can fit a large punching balloon over the mouth of the jug and watch it expand as the yeast exhales carbon dioxide into it!

A hydrometer is a very useful tool for brewing. It measures the specific gravity of the wort (wort=liquid before fermenting) and then the finished brew. In simple terms, it tells you how much sugar (read: potential alcohol) is in the wort, and then after the brew has finished fermenting, it tells you what percentage alcohol it has. This is really only necessary for serious brewers, and I have made numerous batches without using one.

Brushes for cleaning. Most herbalists have the tiny brushes to clean out their tincture bottles. These are great for the airlocks and stoppers. But, you will also need to find a bigger brush to scrub the inside of the jugs and beer bottles. Find one with a long enough handle to reach the bottom of your jug. Kitchen stores might have these, but all brew stores keep a good variety on hand.

A scale is also great to have on hand. In my opinion, no kitchen is complete without some type of scale!

Bottles are another consideration. In such small batches, it is easiest to find some Grolsch-style swing-top bottles that don't require any bottle capping device. There are some breweries still bottling in these, and sometimes it is the same price as buying the empty bottles!

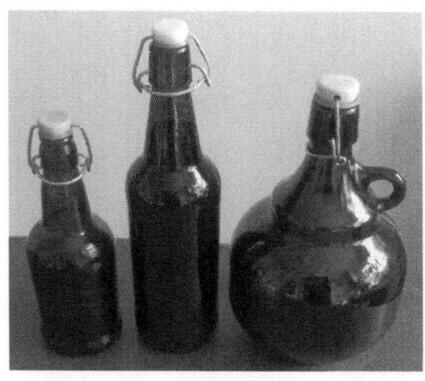

Another option is to save up a lot of beer bottles from friends.  Clean and sterilize them really well.  Then borrow or rent a bottle capper, buy some caps, and cap them.  If you don't already have this stuff or know someone who does, it seems a bit superfluous for such a small batch of beer.

The size of your bottle is a consideration.  If you are brewing medicinal strength, you might only be drinking eight ounces at a time.  Another nice thing about these swing-top bottles is that they do a good job of holding the carbonation once opened, so you could get by with bottling in a 16 ounce and getting two doses out of it.  If you are brewing a milder strength beer for a crowd, it is pure joy to bottle in a 64 ounce "growler", as shown on the far right of the previous picture.

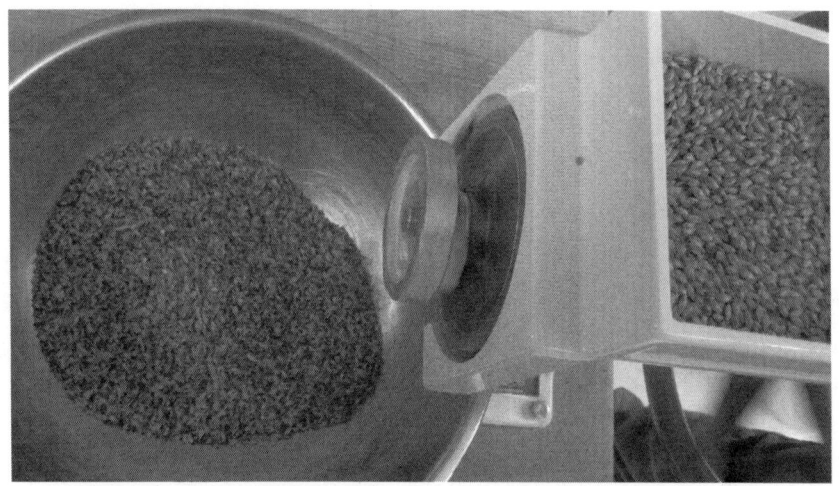
*If you have a flour mill, you can crush your own malt. Just use a coarse setting.*

# INGREDIENTS

**Grains-** Brewing grains are malted, or: sprouted, dried, then roasted. The malting process is what gives beer its characteristic flavor. A particularly good book for growing your own grains and malting them is The Homebrewer's Garden.

By far the most used grain is barley, and can be purchased in a wide gradient of colors from light to dark. Barley must be crushed as close to brewing time as possible to preserve optimum flavor. This can be done with a flour mill, on a very coarse setting, so that each grain is cracked into a few pieces. If you live near a brewing store, they can do this for you.

Other grains are hard to find malted. If you are on a gluten-free diet, I recommend using brown rice syrup or sorghum extract. A bit of roasted millet, amaranth, or buckwheat can be added for additional depth of flavor. On page 24, my instructions for gluten free beer are detailed with lots of photographs.

**Extracts**- These are the liquid syrups extracted from barley malt. They are also available in a range of darkness. Extracts are much simpler to use, especially when formulating herbal beers. They allow you to focus on the herbal formula, require less equipment, and all but eliminate the need for straining. That being said, most homebrewers these days scoff at all extract brews. But the goal here is to make delicious herbal medicine, not beer for purists! Barley malt extract can be bought at most grocery stores in the baking section, usually with the molasses and honey. This is a light variety, and has produced fine ales for me in the past.

Extracts are also available in powder form, called DME, or Dry Malt Extract. It has a longer shelf life, and can be substituted for the liquid equally. If the liquid syrup does ever grow something on top, it is fine to skim off the growth and use what's left. Nothing will grow within the extract itself.

**Bittering agents-** Hops was only introduced to the brewing process in 1000 A.D. That means for about 5000 years, herbs were heavily relied on to bitter beer. And there are just so many wonderful bitter herbs all around us! My personal favorite is fresh dandelion leaves. They are abundant, and I like to think that their liver tonic properties ameliorate any possible damage being done by the alcohol.

I usually choose a bitter herb that corresponds with the needs of an herbal formula. Wormwood would be excellent if a digestive is needed. Horehound would be great in a cough formula. And yarrow would be an excellent choice if there is excess heat, bleeding, or hormonal imbalance involved.

I like to add hops sometimes, too. It does add a nice complexity of flavor, and is perfect for cases of insomnia or disturbed sleep if consumed before bed. However, in excess, hops can contribute to depression, so keep this in mind when formulating.

**Yeast-** In ancient times, brewers depended on the yeast around them to inoculate their brews. Beer was left fermenting in open vessels, attracting the airborne yeasts. Each local wild yeast variety produced different flavors. When a favorite was discovered, they would carve a fresh birch branch with dimples and add it to the fermenting brew. The yeasts were attracted to the sugars in the fresh wood, so they burrowed in and stayed until ready to inoculate the next batch. In Mesopotamia, clay brewing vessels have been unearthed, which have grooves scraped out of the inner pot. This gave the yeast a place live and grow with each new batch of beer, thus ensuring each batch would be as good as the last!

You can still harvest wild yeast today, and I have done so with much success. The reason I started using commercial yeast was simply that of dependability. Wild yeast is a gamble, and when I brew 5 gallon batches, I don't like to risk it!

The types of yeast available is overwhelming. I tend to favor Trappist Ale, Scottish Ale, and English Ale types, but it really depends on the type of beer you want to finish with. These modern yeasts can still be used over and over again. See page 20 for how to do it.

The dry yeast is for the most part, gluten free. Safale US-05 the the most commonly used gluten free yeast. You'll probably have to order this. Even if using the yeast that comes as a liquid, once you add it to your wort, you come out with about 0.5-5 pmm gluten. In order for a product to be labelled gluten free in the United States, it must be below 20 ppm.

**Fruits-** I think the addition of fruits and berries compliment the flavor of herbs quite nicely. If you are experimenting with wild yeasts, don't wash your berries, that white film on the skin is yeast! Add them into the fermentation jug once everything is cooled, and don't cook them first either. However, if you are using commercial yeast, you don't want the wild yeast competing with your strain, so fruit will have to be added to the wort. Add them right after you take it off the heat and have strained any hops or herbs out, so the delicate flavors of the fruit is not compromised, but they get hot enough to kill any living beasties on them. My favorite fresh or frozen fruits are blueberries, raspberries, and blackberries. You can dump the berries right into the fermentation jug, or strain them first.

I should also mention that I use a lot of dried fruits and berries in my herbal formulas, such as jujube, lycii, prunes, and dates. I add these along with the herbs.

**Herbs-** The herbs suitable for beer making are seemingly endless. I usually prepare the herbs just as if I were making a big batch of medicinal strength infusion or decoction (page 25). The herbs you use will be guided by your health needs, what's in season, and what tastes good to you. Make a tea from your intended formula at the same concentration. If it tastes good as a tea, it will taste better as a beer! More on herbal formulation on page 31.

## A word about straining ingredients

If you don't have two large pots to strain back and forth in, or you can't be bothered, you can throw all of the ingredients into a large muslin bag. Or a pillowcase! Keep the top of the bag clothes-pinned to the top of the pot so you can easily add ingredients throughout the process. You might consider also having a smaller muslin bag for adding those final delicate herbs or hops after the other ingredients have been removed.

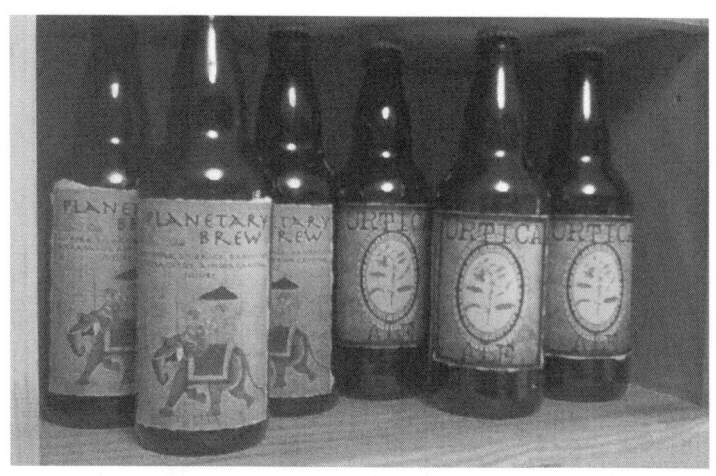

## KEEPING IT CLEAN

**Sterilizing Your Equipment-** There are a lot of sanitizers on the market that are specifically made for the homebrewer. The one I have always used with good results is called B Brite. It sterilizes through oxygenation. If you get a build up of gunk on your equipment, it will clean that, too.

Some dishwashers have a sanitize setting, but be sure to scrub the inside of all equipment with something like B Brite that will dissolve build up. And rinse really well.

Everything that comes into contact with a pre-ferment brew (wort), must be completely sterile. That means spoons, strainers, hydrometer (if your using one), airlocks, etc. No need to sterilize the pots or anything that will be used in the boiling process. The heat will sterilize that stuff. Also, after the batch has finished fermenting, all of the bottling equipment will need to be sterilized.

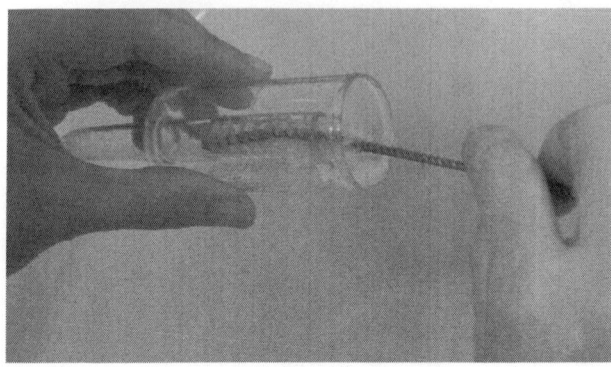

*Cleaning the airlock*

**My technique-** My first year working in a microbiology lab, I was the grunt, cleaning and sterilizing glassware. Needless to say, I developed a technique!

The first thing I do is fill a sink with hot, soapy water. I use Dr. Bronner's brand soap because it is so easy to rinse clean. Everything gets a good scrub, inside and out with the brushes. I have a set of

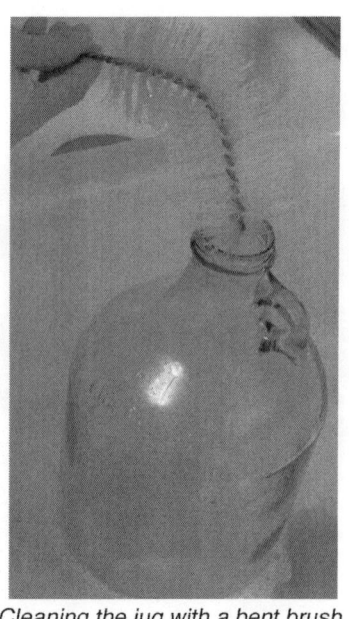

*Cleaning the jug with a bent brush*

different size brushes to fit into even the small airlock holes. The really big brushes for the jugs can be bent to fit the shape of the inside of any container perfectly. Then everything gets rinsed. And rinsed again. And once more for good measure.

Now, I put a couple of teaspoons of sanitizer (or according to package directions) in a jug and fill it with warm water. Then let it set for thirty minutes and funnel it into the other jug and repeat. Once the second jug is finished, I pour the same sanitizer water into a small, very clean sink or bowl with all of my other equipment that needs to be sterile: airlocks, funnel, strainer, stoppers, and a hydrometer, and let these soak in the solution for thirty minutes.. Everything gets rinsed 5 or six times as soon as the sanitizer is drained from it. Rinsing is the key. So rinse with fury, pour a few cups of water into the jug and slosh and spin and shake, then dump and repeat.

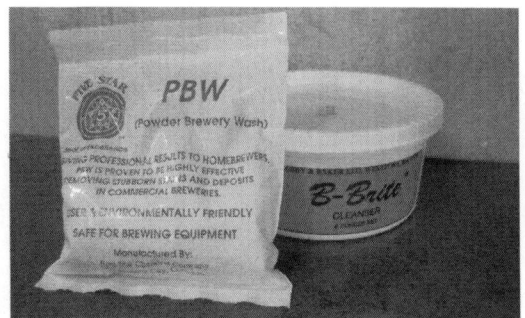

*Some commercially available cleaners.*

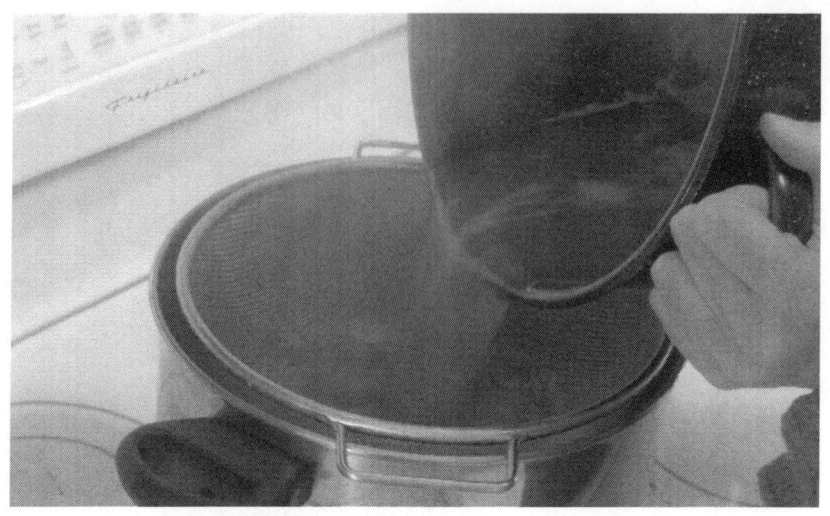

## BREWING STAGES

Below is an outline of the steps required to brew, and what is happening behind the scenes in the yeast world.

**Wort-** The first stage in the brewing process is preparing the wort. At this stage, the correct level of sugar is added to the wort for proper yeast activity. Too much sugar will give you a possibly sweeter, and more alcoholic brew. Too little sugar will result in incomplete fermentation with low alcohol. This is where a hydrometer comes in handy. But, if you follow these recipes, you should be fine. If you find a recipe for a bigger batch, just scale it down proportionally to fit your brew size.

**Pitching the Yeast-** The next stage of brewing is pitching the yeast. This is done when the wort is 70°, which is the optimal temperature for yeast development. Before adding the yeast, it helps to oxygenate the brew with a whisk, since yeast need oxygen for their metabolism.

There are several ways to pitch yeast. Dry yeast can be pitched right into the wort. Some folks prefer to make a yeast starter culture by feeding the yeast some boiled and cooled sugar water, and waiting until the yeast become active to add it. Follow the same directions as below for storing leftover yeast, only instead of refrigerating it, let it become active by leaving it at about 70° overnight. This requires an airlock and sanitized equipment, and really adds an extra step for our medicine-making purposes.

My favorite yeast is made by Wyeast. They come in mylar packets, with an internal pouch that you have to smack to release the yeast into the nutrients. Once the mylar bag swells up, you know it is ready to pitch.

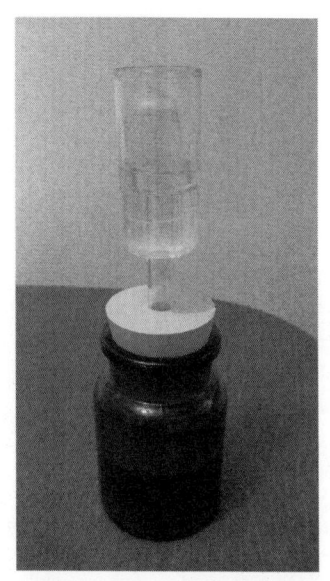
*A tiny yeast culture before going into the fridge.*

No matter what method you use, only use 1/4-1/2 of

the yeast in a packet that is intended for 5 gallon batches. Remaining yeast can be cultured by boiling 3 cups of water and 1/2 Cup of sugar. Add this to a sterile bottle with an airlock, and cool to 70°. Add the yeast and refrigerate. Then, when you are ready to brew just take it out of the refrigerator and let it set at 70° overnight before pitching. Dry yeast can be left in the package and put in the freezer. It usually keeps just fine for a few weeks.

**Fermentation-** Okay, you have pitched your yeast and placed your airlocks on your fermenting vessels. Now you rig whatever you can to keep the temperature as close to 70° as possible. If it is a little cooler, just allow for longer fermentation time. If it is a little warmer, it will go faster. Keep a thermometer next to it to monitor the temperature. In the winter, you could keep it near a radiator or wood stove. In the summer, ancient cultures would bury their brew in the ground to keep it cool! One option would be to place the fermentation vessel into an unglazed terra cotta pot and pack it with sand. Moisten the sand, and there you have it. This is based on the Zeer Pot, and works by evaporative cooling.

During fermentation, the yeast are consuming the sugar and oxygen, and converting it into carbon dioxide and alcohol. At a certain point, either the sugar will run out, or the alcohol will become too concentrated and will kill the yeast. Wait until there are no more bubbles in the brew, and the airlock is no longer gurgling. You want fermentation to stop completely before bottling, or you will have some minor explosions with glass shard shrapnel. Trust me.

It may take a day or two before your brew gets really active. And each one occurs differently. In my experience, gluten-free beers never really go crazy with activity. So long as you see some nice bubbling action in the airlocks, and notice it taper off at some point, rest assured. Fermentation has happened.

**Priming and Bottling-** So the fermentation is complete, now it is time to bottle! The first thing to do is prepare a bit of priming sugar to feed the hungry yeast while they are trapped in a sealed bottle, creating natural carbonation (unlike modern beer, which is pumped with carbon dioxide after the yeast has been killed off). Priming is detailed on page 27.

Once your priming sugar is ready, put it into the bottom of your bottling bucket. This is just a pot or bucket that will be a temporary vessel to get your brew from the fermentation vessel to the bottle. And, you guessed it, it must be sanitized!

Now very gently pour or siphon the brew into the bottling bucket. The idea here is to get the brew without any of the yeast sediment, called dregs, that lies at the bottom.  And don't oxygenate too much!

At this stage, most brewers are very careful to avoid oxygenating the brew, and would never pour.  They only siphon.  The reason is, oxygenation produces off flavors.  Though, with medicinal beer, it is really okay.  I would just be gentle with it in order to not over-activate the yeast.  Or find yourself some food grade clear tubing and learn to siphon.  It's handy.

**Siphoning-** all you need to do is elevate the full vessel a few feet above the empty vessel.  Kitchen counters work great for this.  Next, have a good friend place one end of the tube into the fermentation vessel (on the kitchen counter), just above the dregs.  Now place the bottling bucket on the floor below.  Take the other (lowest) end of the tube and suck until the brew flows down freely.  You will get a good sneak preview of the flavor of your brew!  Repeat this with the other jug, putting both into the same bottling bucket.  Make sure you always keep the tube above the dregs.  You can put your thumb over the end to stop the flow.

There are lots of siphoning equipment options out there that eliminate the need to have two people, or use your mouth.  But where is the fun in that?  But seriously, if you really get into this, invest in some siphoning equipment.  The kind I use has a pumping action at the top to get the siphon started.  I added a bottle siphoning wand as well. It automatically stops siphoning when you lift the tube out of the vessel you are siphoning into, via a spring-loaded valve. This entire siphoning setup is under $20, and will save you a lot of spills and reduce the possibility of contamination.

So now we need to get the primed brew from the bottling bucket into some sterilized bottles. If you don't have a siphoning setup, you can (gently!) funnel it in, waiting a bit for the foam to go down, and adding more. Or, use the siphoning method described above. If you're just using tubing, use your thumb to stop the flow from the tube before moving to the next bottle. You might want to put the bottle you are filling into a pan or bucket, so you can catch anything that might flow over.

It is a good idea to leave some head room. About 1 inch of space should be left in each bottle. Not enough headspace results in an uncarbonated beer. Too much headspace can over-oxygenate the yeast and lead to exploding bottles.

Cap off your bottles, and wait about 2 weeks for full carbonation. Flavors will mellow with time, but this living brew is best in its first six months of life.

Store in a cool place.

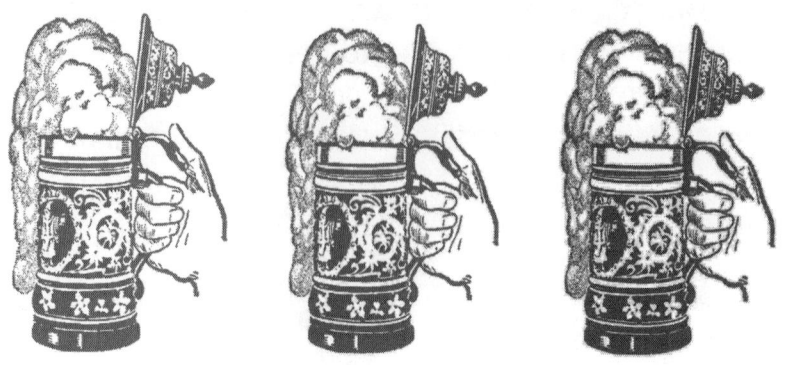

## INSTRUCTIONS FOR THREE TYPES OF BREWING

**Extract Brewing-** Refers to brewing with only the liquid or powdered extracts. This is the simplest method, and I think most suited for the brewer who is not necessarily interested in investing in equipment. It is simply a matter of making a big batch of herbal tea, straining, and adding your extract. Below is the step-by-step process with photographs:

1. Prepare your "tea".

You can either add your herbs directly to the water and then strain through a sieve, or just brew the herbs in a straining bag and pull the bag out to avoid pouring such a large pot of water.

For roots, bark, twigs, dried fruit, and thick, coarse leaves, a decoction is in order. Add the herbs to the pot with 1.5 gallons of water. Cover and simmer (never boil rapidly) for about 30 minutes.

For flowers and leaves, make an infusion by boiling the water, turning off the heat, and adding the herbs. Cover the pot and steep 30 minutes.

If there are both infusing herbs and decocting herbs, then I will simmer the roots, covered, for about 30 minutes, then turn off the heat and add the infusing herbs for thirty minutes, covered. If you are wanting to extract volatile oils from certain herbs like peppermint or lemon balm, add these to the wort after turning the heat off, and letting them steep, covered, as it cools before straining into the jugs.

If you have your own favorite technique for making herbal teas, by all means, go for it! Some Chinese formulas brew for hours, and some infusions are best left overnight. Have fun and experiment with this!

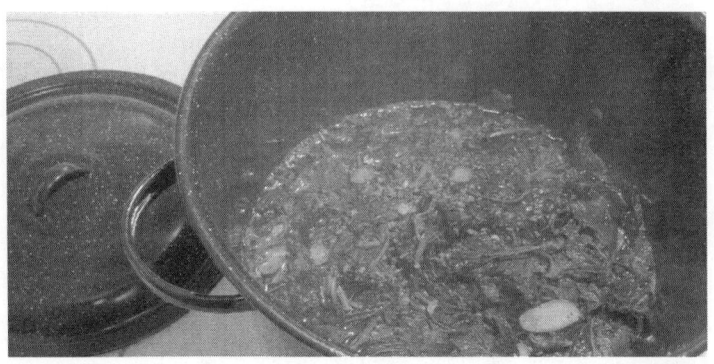

2. Strain the herbs (or remove the straining bag) and add the extract of your choice, according to the recipe. Bring to a gentle boil, and add a couple of tablespoons of hops in a muslin bag if you are using any. Simmer for 40 minutes uncovered.

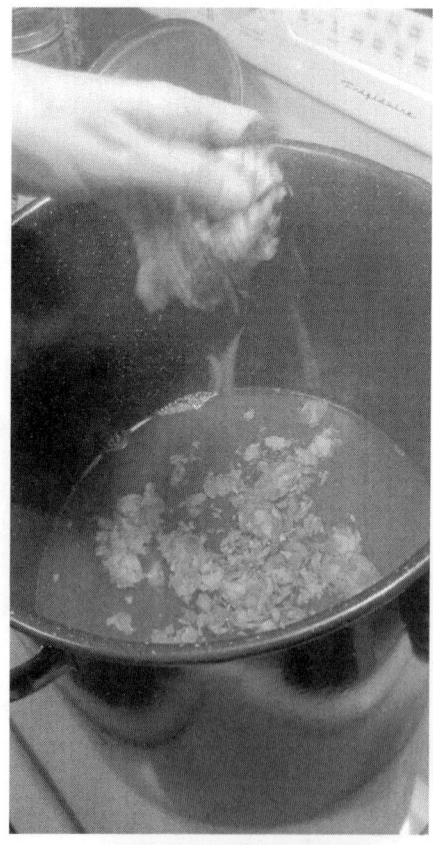
*Hopping the wort.*

3. Allow to cool to 70°. The faster you can bring the wort to 70º, the better your brew will taste. You can do this by preparing a cold water bath in your kitchen sink and placing the pot in. Just don't let it get cooler than 70º. Aerate the wort with a whisk, because yeast love oxygen! Funnel into the sanitized jugs, dividing the wort equally. There should be plenty of head room in each jug since it might become quite active and frothy. Add your yeast according to package directions. I usually only add 1/4 of the package to each jug.

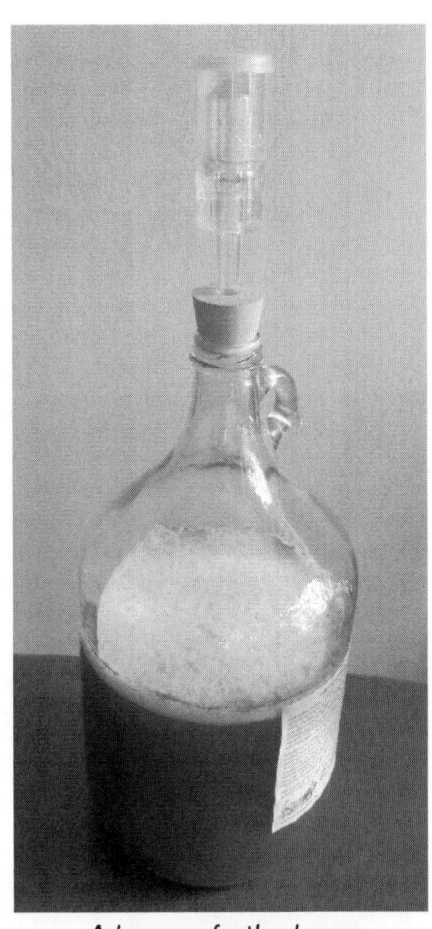
*A happy, frothy brew after 24-48 hours.*

4. Place the airlock into the rubber stopper, and place it into the mouth of the jug so that it is airtight. Fill the airlock with water to the fill line and place the cap on it. Allow to ferment at about 70° until all bubbling stops completely (7-10 days).

5. Once all activity has ceased, it is time to prime! Priming just means feeding the yeast, so that they will naturally ferment the beer once an airtight cap is in place to hold in the carbon dioxide. Boil about 1/2 Cup of water with 3 tablespoons (or 1.5 oz) sugar for every gallon of finished beer and pour this into a sanitized pot or bucket large enough to hold the contents of both jugs (roughly 1.5 gallons). Then pour or siphon the jugs into this vessel, leaving behind the sludge (called

dregs) at the bottom. Save these dregs, they can be used for many things, see page 51.

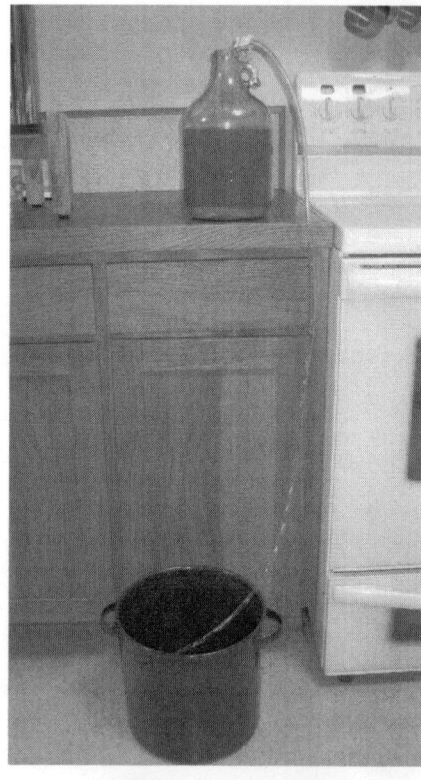
*A siphoning setup.*

6. Now siphon or pour this brew into some sterilized Grolsch style swing-top bottles and place the caps on. I have seen some folks pour the brew back into the original jugs after cleaning them. This is risky, because these jugs aren't made to withstand the pressure of naturally carbonated fluids. And if it becomes over-carbonated, it will explode.

Your beer will be ready to drink in two weeks!

**All Grain Brewing-** This is very similar to the extract brewing method above, except you'll be adding malted grain as the only form of sugar. As far as I know, there is no gluten free malted grain available, so those with gluten intolerance should stick with the extract brewing.

Follow all of the steps above, replacing step 2 with the following:

Strain the herbs (or remove the straining bag). Place malted grain in a muslin bag and place it in the herbal tea you have prepared. Clip the bag to the pot, so that it is open, as shown. This allows the grain some elbow room. Slowly bring this up to 150°, uncovered. Remove from heat, cover, and let sit for one hour.

If you are using hops, place a tablespoon or two into a small bag and toss it into the strained wort. Bring to a boil, and simmer uncovered for 60 minutes.

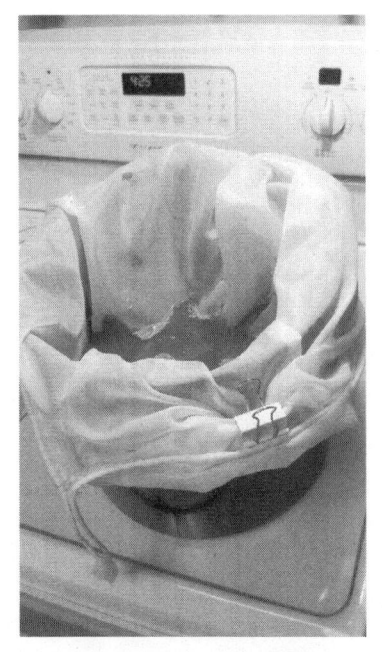

Continue to Step 3 on page 26.

*The malted grains in the straining bag, clipped to the pot.*

**Partial Mash Brewing-** This simply refers to recipes that use both grains and extracts. If you want to use an extract, but still want some fresh malted flavors, this might be something to experiment with.

Below are the outlined steps:

1. Make your herbal tea formula, as indicated in step 1, page 24.

2. Strain the herbs. Place the malted grain in a muslin bag and tie it off or clip it to the pot as shown on previous page. Slowly bring this up to 150°, uncovered. Remove from heat, cover, and let sit for one hour. Strain the mash (malted grain) off, or remove the bag. Add the extract and hops, if your using any and bring to the boil again. Simmer for 40 minutes, uncovered.

Continue with step 3, page 26.

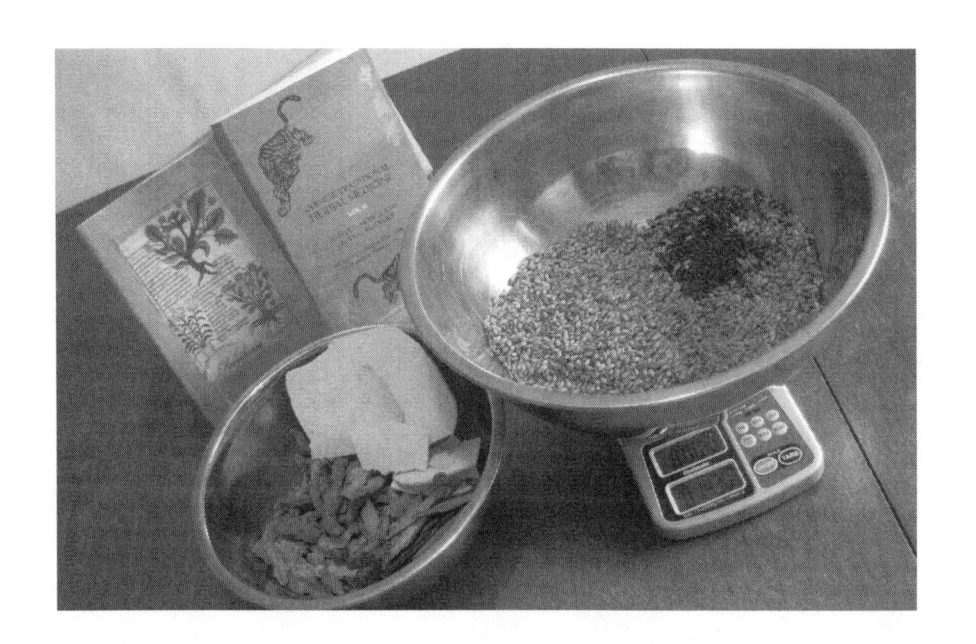

## CUSTOM HERBAL FORMULAS

This is the fun part! There are so many variations and possibilities regarding what kind of herbal formula you choose. So, let's start with the first question: What are your favorite herbs? For your first batch, I say you just use whatever your favorite tea may be. You can even use pre-made herbal tea blends! I would avoid tea bags, though. They just aren't going to be economical when making up such a large pot of tea. Besides, I like for my herbs to be unrestrained in the tea as I brew them. It makes a big difference.

After your first batch of your favorite tea-based brew, then you can begin experimenting with other flavors and intentions.

The next question is: How strong do you want your medicine? If you want it at full medicinal strength, you should be careful to observe proper dosage, which is usually one cup (as in, 8 ounces), three times a day. If you want it to be more of a casual beverage that you can drink an entire bottle of, or share among friends, you will want to decrease the amount of herbs you add. If you are making a digestive to drink with a meal, you might want 12 ounces. But, if this is going to be a nightcap to help you sleep, you probably don't want to consume too much fluids right before bed.

Another consideration when deciding what amount of herb to use is simply the strength of each herb. Advanced herbalists will be familiar with proper dosage for the herbs they are working with. However, if you are just starting out in the world of herbs, look through a few different herb books to get an idea of proper dosage.

There are many schools of thought regarding what is considered "medicinal strength". For me, it is up to one ounce of herb for each pint of water. That concentration is more in line with Eastern medicine making. This will prove to be a very strong concoction, and I love them this way.

For those starting out in this new adventure, you might want to try something like one ounce per quart of water. Do a trial run. Try making a quart of tea at this concentration, following the instructions on page 24, and then adjust it how you see fit. Keep trying until you get it right. This is the easiest part, so it's best to get it right before you begin your brew.

So, once you have decided how strong you want your brew, and selected your favorite herbs, how do you put them all together? The first thing you do is come up with a total weight of herbs to use in a 1.5 gallon batch. For a casual beer that I want to drink with friends, I will use 6 ounces of dried herbs total . Then I choose the herb with the main "action" or flavor that I am trying to achieve. Let's look at my Nettles Spring Tonic Ale, page 40. In this recipe, nettles is the featured, or <u>main</u> herb. It's actions are diuretic and tonic, which is perfect for cleansing winter stagnation. It's flavor is slightly acrid and sweet.

Burdock root, dandelion leaf, and blueberries are the <u>supporting</u> herbs in this formula, which means they support the actions of nettles. Orange peel acts as an <u>assisting</u> herb, meaning that it enhances the actions of the main and supporting herbs. In this case, orange peel dries dampness and helps keep this heavily tonic formula from causing stagnation.

Lastly, you have the <u>conducting</u> herbs. These herbs direct the formula to a particular organ system, or coax their properties to move in a certain direction in the body. In this case, fresh ginger and licorice are the conducting herbs. Fresh ginger is warming, and will help circulate the formula throughout the body. Licorice is harmonizing. This means that when included in a formula, it smoothes out the flavors and actions so that all of the herbs are working together. It directs the formula to the spleen and stomach. I include fresh ginger and dried licorice root in almost all of my beer formulas. They taste wonderful, and are usually the perfect conducting herbs.

To summarize, each formula should have 1-3 herbs that work together in flavor and action, and are used in the highest concentration. These are considered the main herbs. Next, you have a few herbs that support the actions of the main herb(s), and are used in lower quantity. Then, you have assisting herbs, which address other symptoms or generally enhance the overall formula. Lastly, the conducting herbs will take the formula where you want it to go. Assisting and conducting herbs are usually used in the smallest ratios.

Here is a general example of a formula. We want to finish with 6 ounces of dried herb, so to make it easy, I am dividing the formula into 6 parts.

## Main Herbs-3 parts
## Supporting Herbs-2 parts
## Conducting Herbs-1 part

As you can see, you don't need to include all four categories in a formula. This is simply a way of bringing balance and symmetry to your brew. While this is an ancient formulation strategy, there are many others. Each herbalist has their own, and this one is just mine. I have found it to suit the brewing process well, so give it a try!

I should note that most of the herbs I use in my recipes are considered by most to be "Chinese". The herbs commonly used by Chinese Medicine practitioners happen to taste very good in beer. And as my teacher, Michael Tierra, likes to say "Any herb can be a Chinese herb, it just depends on how you use it."

To me, roots and bark tend to taste better in brew recipes. Anything with a lot of volatile oils tends to overpower the rest of the formula. But that is simply a matter of taste.

I recommend that if you don't know the herbs you are using really well, try using a formula written by an established herbalist. I have always enjoyed Rosemary Gladstar's recipes, for instance.

## A WORD ON THE ENERGY OF BEER

In all ancient herbal disciplines, the energy and flavor of an herb is of utmost importance. While they all differ slightly in the number of flavors they recognize, or what has a warming or cooling energy, they have plenty in common.

According to Traditional Chinese Medicine (since that is my focus in study), any type of alcohol is warming, sweet, bitter, and toxic.* It is used to improve blood circulation, conduct medicine through the body, and disperse cold.

The color of the beer also effects the energetics of it. The darkness of the malt represents the level of roasting the grain has undergone. Since roasting adds warmth, the darker the beer, the warmer the energy. It is good to keep this in mind, as you might want to alter the recipes according to the energy you are trying to attain. If someone has a warm to hot condition, Use the palest malt with cooling herbs such as mint, nettles, burdock, and meadowsweet. Heat signs are red skin, feelings of heat, dryness, dark urine, constipation, or anxiety.

Signs of cold are paleness, general coldness, edema (swelling), diarrhea, infertility, and fatigue. With these signs, you want to use a darker beer, like a porter or stout. Use warming herbs like ginger, cayenne, sassafras, and yerba mansa.

*The toxic aspect of alcohol is only in large doses, of course. The Chinese culture has a long history of using alcohol for medicine. In fact, the Chinese character for doctor literally translates to "wine shaman"!

# Recipes

This is a list of my personal favorite brews that I have crafted over the years. Each one is a particular style of brew, strength of medicinal qualities, and darkness of malts. These aspects are discussed briefly after each recipe, along with ideas on how you can customize them to fit your needs.

Be creative, but most importantly, be confident! This stuff is hard to mess up. The only time I have had a beer go wrong was my very first batch. My professor of microbiology in college led the class in a beer-making activity. With thousands of dollars worth of equipment, sanitizers, and bottles, we created a beer that was flat and lifeless. With my pots and jugs, this has yet to happen.

# ALL EXTRACT BREWS

The next couple of recipes are simple to convert to gluten-free. All you need to do is omit the Barley Malt Extract. In its place, use the following:

**28 oz (2 cups) Sorghum Malt Extract**
**4 oz (1/3 Cup) Brown Rice Syrup**

Everything else is exactly the same!

This brew will not become as active as the barley extract beers. Gluten-free beers will also have less head when poured. So, if you notice these things, just know it is the character of this type of beer, and you did everything perfectly!

Sorghum beer is actually preferred over barley beers in many parts of Africa. The brown rice syrup just adds a bit of something extra, but you could omit that and replace it with honey, maple syrup, or more sorghum.

# GENERAL RECIPE

*Follow these guidelines to brew your own, custom beer using the pure extract method. Use your favorite purchased herbal blend, or create your own!*

## Light on the Herbs

*If you want a beer that you can drink by the bottle-full, and share freely at parties, use these concentrations of herbs. Just be sure to use herbs that you wouldn't mind drinking a big pot of tea of.*

**1.5 Gallons Filtered Water**
**1-1.5 lbs Fresh Herbs Total**
   **-OR-**
**6-9 oz Dried Herbs Total**

## Medicinal Strength

*These are higher doses, which means you will consume smaller amounts at a time. Still, be sure to really know your herbs, both in flavor, and in medicinal intensity.*

**1.5 Gallons Filtered Water**
**2-3 lbs Fresh Herbs Total**
   **-OR-**
**9-15 oz Dried Herbs Total**

## Extracts

*The more extract you use, the higher the alcohol content will tend to be. Somewhere in this range has always worked for me.*

**22-28 oz Extract, Liquid or Dry**

# NETTLES SPRING ALE

*This is my favorite Spring tonic! It is a light, all extract brew. Although the herbs are added in medicinal-strength quantity, they are tonic and gentle.
So enjoy by the bottle-full!
Harvest stinging nettles when they are about 6 inches tall. I only harvest and use the top 4-6 leaves.*

**1.5 Gallons Filtered Water**
**1.5 lbs Fresh Nettle Tops**
**3 oz Fresh Dandelion Leaves**
**1.5 oz Dried Burdock Root**
**1 oz Dried Orange Peel**
**½ oz Fresh Ginger, Thinly Sliced**
**½ oz Dried Licorice Root**

**2 Tablespoons Centennial Hops**
**22 oz Light Barley Malt Extract**

**10 oz Blueberries, Fresh or Frozen**

**¼- ½ Package London Ale Yeast**

1. Place herbs in 1.5 gallons of water in a large pot. Bring just to boil, simmer 30 minutes, covered. Strain out the herbs.
2. Add extract syrup and hops and return to the boil, and simmer for 40 minutes. Remove from heat and strain hops out.
3. Add blueberries while the wort cools to 70°.
4. Once wort reaches 70°, strain out the berries, pour into jugs, and pitch the yeast, as described on page 26.

# YI SHENG'S BREW

*In China, scientists analyzed ancient pottery that once held fermented beverages. All of the herbs in this brew were found in traces on the ancient pottery.*
*This is a light, all extract brew.*
*The concentration of herbs is light, so it would be a wonderful beverage to bring to a party for immediate conversation!*

**1.5 Gallons Filtered Water**
**6 oz Dried Hawthorn Fruits**
**4 oz Jujube Fruits (aka Red Dates)**

**22 oz Light Barley Malt Extract**
**6 oz Brown Rice Syrup**

**¼- ½ Package Whitbread Ale Yeast**

**½ Cup Jasmine**
**½ Cup Chrysanthemum**

1. Place the hawthorn and jujube in 1.5 gallons of water in a large pot. Bring just to boil, simmer 30 minutes, covered. Strain out the herbs.
2. Add extract syrup and return to the boil, and simmer for 40 minutes. Remove from heat.
3. Allow wort to cool to 70°.
4. Pour into jugs, and pitch the yeast, as described on page 26.
5. Once activity has ceased, add the jasmine and chrysanthemum equally to the brewing jugs, stirring to moisten them, and allow to infuse for two days before bottling. The flowers will float, so that will make avoiding them during siphoning easy.

# ALL GRAIN BREWS

These are great fun to experiment with, and really quite easy when brewing in small batches. If you do decide to increase your batch size, you will need some serious upgrades in equipment, though.

Experiment with different colors of barley, according to your taste...

# GENERAL RECIPE

*Follow these guidelines to brew your own custom beer using pure malted grains as the sugar. Use your favorite purchased herbal blend, or create your own!*

## Light on the Herbs
*If you want a beer that you can drink by the bottle-full, and share freely at parties, use these concentrations of herbs. Just be sure to use herbs that you wouldn't mind drinking a big pot of tea of.*

**2 Gallons Filtered Water**
**1-1.5 lbs Fresh Herbs Total**
   **-OR-**
**6-9 oz Dried Herbs Total**

## Medicinal Strength
*These are higher doses, which means you will consume smaller amounts at a time. Still, be sure to really know your herbs, both in flavor, and in medicinal intensity.*

**2 Gallons Filtered Water**
**2-3 lbs Fresh Herbs Total**
   **-OR-**
**9-15 oz Dried Herbs Total**

## Grains
*You probably already know what kind of beer you like. If you like it dark, up to half dark or chocolate malt. But, always maintain the majority of your grains to be pale. If you really want the flavor of your herbs to come through, keep it lighter.*

**2.5 lbs Crushed Malted Barley**

# SECOND TREASURE TONIC

*This is a very tasty, warming, strong medicinal herbal brew. I drink a cup of it at a time, three times a day when I need it. This recipe is for a light ale, but it is also wonderful with some dark, chocolatey malts. It's a qi tonic, so if you're vital energy is feeling drained, try this brew!*

**2 Gallons Filtered Water**
**5 oz Jujube Fruit (Red Date)**
**3 oz Panax Ginseng**
**2 oz Astragalus Root**
**2 oz Cinnamon Twig**
**1.5 oz Fresh Ginger, Thinly Sliced**
**1 oz Dried Licorice Root**

**2 lb Crushed Pale Ale (light) Malt**
**½ lb Munich Malt**
**2T Cascade Hops**

**¼- ½ Package American Ale Yeast**

1. Place the herbs in 2 gallons of water in a large pot. Bring just to boil, simmer 30 minutes, covered. Strain out the herbs.
2. Follow instructions on page 28 for boiling and straining the grains.
3. Allow wort to cool to 70°.
4. Pour into jugs, and pitch the yeast, as described on page 26.

# PLANETARY PORTER

*I made this beer as a tribute to my teachers, Michael and Lesley Tierra, who have spent their lives healing with and teaching about the planet's herbs.
It's a semi-dark beer, and is a very lovely beer to share with a crowd by the bottle-full.*

**2 Gallons Filtered Water**
**½ lb Fresh Nettles, or 3 oz Dried Nettles**
**2 oz Eleuthero Root**
**One Handful Fresh Dandelion Leaves**
**1 oz Ashwagandha**
**½ oz Dried Licorice Root**
**1 oz Hawthorn Fruit**

**1.5 lb Crushed Pale Ale Malt**
**1 lb Crushed Chocolate Malt**
**2T Cascade Hops**

**¼- ½ Package Scottish Ale Yeast**

1. Place the herbs in 2 gallons of water in a large pot. Bring just to boil, simmer 30 minutes, covered. Strain out the herbs.
2. Follow instructions on page 28 for boiling and straining the grains.
3. Allow wort to cool to 70°.
4. Pour into jugs, and pitch the yeast, as described on page 26.

# DANDELION STOUT

*This is one of my favorite simple blends. I got the idea when I started making my herbal coffee substitute from these roots. It is another good one to share and drink freely. Well, you know, to a point.*

**2 Gallons Filtered Water**
**3 oz Roasted Dandelion Root***
**2 oz Roasted Burdock Root***
**1 oz Roasted Chicory Root***

**1.5 lb Crushed Pale Ale Malt**
**½ lb Chocolate Malt**
**½ lb Black Malt**
**2T Eroica Hops**

**¼- ½ Package Irish Ale Yeast**

1. Place the herbs in 2 gallons of water in a large pot. Bring just to boil, simmer 30 minutes, covered. Strain out the herbs.
2. Follow instructions on page 28 for boiling and straining the grains.
3. Allow wort to cool to 70°.
4. Pour into jugs, and pitch the yeast, as described on page 26.

- *For instructions on roasting these roots, see page 57.*

# PARTIAL MASH BREWS

These are the most common types of recipes for homebrewers you will find. Always use a pale ale malt extract for your base, and then use the grain malts for whatever darkness and flavor you are trying to achieve.

Any of the all extract brews can be converted to partial mash, just by adding some malted grain for flavor.

# GENERAL RECIPE

*Follow these guidelines to brew your own, custom beer using both extract and malted grains. Use your favorite purchased herbal blend, or create your own!*

### Light on the Herbs

If you want a beer that you can drink by the bottle-full, and share freely at parties, use these concentrations of herbs. Just be sure to use herbs that you wouldn't mind drinking a big pot of tea of.

**1.5 Gallons Filtered Water**
**1-1.5 lbs Fresh Herbs Total**
   **-OR-**
**6-9 oz Dried Herbs Total**

### Medicinal Strength

These are higher doses, which means you will consume smaller amounts at a time. Still, be sure to really know your herbs, both in flavor, and in medicinal intensity.

**1.5 Gallons Filtered Water**
**2-3 lbs Fresh Herbs Total**
   **-OR-**
**9-15 oz Dried Herbs Total**

### Extract & Grains

Stick with a light, or pale extract, and add color and flavor using dark, caramel, chocolate, or black malted grains.

**22-28 oz Malt Extract, Liquid or Dry**
**½ lb Malted Grain**

# ROMAN ALE

*I made this recipe when my husband was doing a lot of studying. Luckily, I had most of these herbs in the garden. It is very light in color, and the perfect relaxation before study (if you drink just a glass.)
Make note! The steps are in different order for this recipe. A good example of how to treat those fragile volatile oil-containing herbs.*

**1.5 Gallons Filtered Water**

**½ lb Caramel Malted Barley**

**24 oz Malt Extract, Liquid or Dry**
**2T Cascade Hops**

**2 oz Dried Borage, or 6 oz Fresh**
**1 oz Rosemary, or 3 oz Fresh**
**½ oz Sage, or 1.5 oz Fresh**
**1 oz Dried Ginkgo Leaves**
**1 oz Dried Gotu Kola**

**¼- ½ Package American Ale Yeast**

1. Follow instructions on page 28 for boiling and straining the GRAINS in 1.5 gallons water.
2. Add extract syrup and hops and return to the boil, and simmer for 40 minutes, uncovered. Remove from heat and strain hops out.
3. Place herbs in a large pot, and pour the wort over them. Cover. Allow to steep 30 minutes. Strain out the herbs and let cool.
4. Once wort reaches 70°, pour into jugs, and pitch the yeast, as described on page 26.

# ELDERBERRY PORTER

*This is a fantastically complex brew. Dark, sweet, and just the thing to keep your immune system strong.
Make note! The steps are in different order for this recipe. You want to add your berries last!*

**1.5 Gallons Filtered Water**
**½ oz Dried Licorice Root**
**1/3 oz Reishi**
**½ lb Dark Chocolate Malt**
**2 T Brambling Cross Hops**

**28 oz Malt Extract, Liquid or Dry**

**2 lbs Mixed Berries, Fresh or Frozen**
    **Elderberry, Blackberry, Raspberry, etc.**

**¼- ½ Package Scottish Ale Yeast**

1. Place the herbs, malted grain, and hops in 1.5 gallons of water in a large pot. Bring slowly to boil, simmer 30 minutes, covered. Strain out the herbs.
2. Add the extract and bring back to the boil. Simmer 40 minutes, uncovered. Remove from heat.
3. Add the berries, and allow the wort to cool to 70°.
4. Pour into jugs, with the berries, and pitch the yeast, as described on page 26°. Allow the wort and fruit to ferment together for 14 days.
5. Siphon both jugs into a bottling bucket with the priming sugar, leaving the berries and dregs behind.
6. Bottle.

# SAVE THE DREGS!

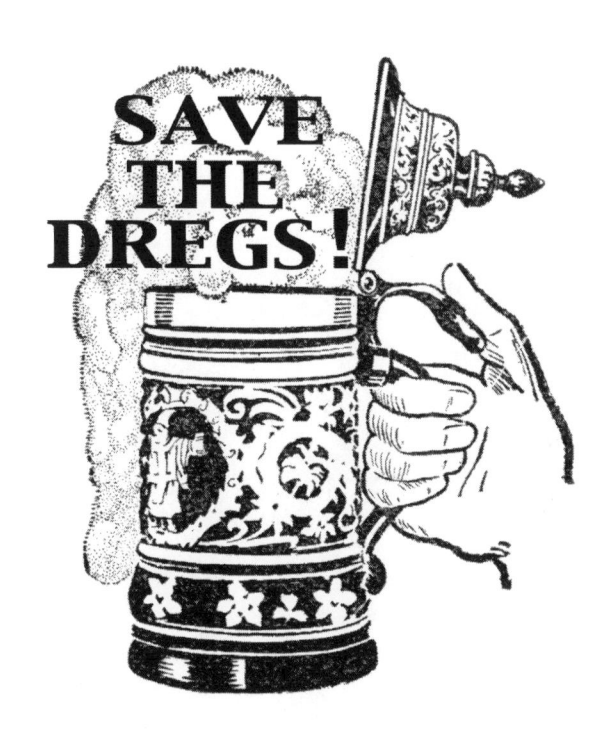

Now that your beautiful beer is made, what do you do with all of that sludge at the bottom? That sludge is called the dregs, and it is like liquid vitamins! Most brewers dump it out and go on with their day. But not us herbalists! We recognize the value of that rich, living, bubbling slurry. It is a great source of the B vitamin complex, proteins, potassium, and chromium.

There are so many ways to make good use of your dregs. It can be as simple as adding a tablespoon to a glass of your favorite beverage. You can use it in a marinade, add some to a jambalaya, or use it to start your next batch of beer! I feed it to my animals by putting some in their water. Even my plants get some!

Since brewing yeast is the same organism as baking yeast, I tend to use it as a sourdough starter. It gets active right away, and as you feed it and use it, the hoppy flavor subsides (but I kinda like that flavor). So below are some of my family's favorite sourdough recipes, beginning with the starter itself. If you have a favorite gluten-free flour mix, just substitute that for the sorghum flour.

# SOURDOUGH STARTER

**1 Cup Beer Dregs
1 Cup Rye Flour, - or -
    Sorghum Flour for Gluten-free Version**

Mix together in a bowl with enough room for the starter to swell and bubble. Leave in a warm place overnight.

The next day, remove a cup, and feed it with ½ cup flour and ½ cup water. You can use the cup that you removed in a recipe, if it seemed fairly active and bubbly already. Leave it in a warm place for another day.

At this point, it should be good to go. If you aren't going to be using it in the next day or two, refrigerate it. Then, when you are ready to use it, just take it out the night before to give it a chance to re-activate.

Keep feeding it with equal parts flour and water as you notice it losing bubbly-ness. Also, each time you feed it, take some off and use it. It is up to you how big of a batch you want to keep going. It needs to be fed every few days. If you can't keep up with it, offer some to friends!

Rye flour is the best sourdough flour there is. The yeast just seem to take to it right away. But, feel free to use any yeast you like.

The gluten-free version doesn't get as bubbly and active, but it really is delicious. Just give it a longer rising time in your recipes.

# SOURDOUGH CREPES

*I have even made sourdough crepes with nothing but watered down sourdough starter, and they are delicious. This version is a bit more sophisticated!*

**1 Cup Sourdough Starter**
**2 Eggs, Beaten**
**¼ tsp Salt**
**1/8 Cup Oil or Butter**
**1/8 Cup Water or Milk**

Whisk all ingredients together. Let sit for 20 minutes.

Heat your griddle on medium heat. When water sizzles and dances around on it, it is ready.

Brush the griddle with some oil. Pour the batter on with a ladle, in a circle pattern, and then use the bottom of the ladle to smooth it out even further. This is a technique, and if this is your first time, don't worry. You'll get better.

The secret is a hot griddle, so don't jump the gun!

My favorite toppings for these are brie, blueberries, and apples. All at once. Yum!

# BROWNIES!

**2-3 T Dutch Cocoa or Carob**
**½ Cup Butter**
**2 Eggs, Beaten**
**1 t Vanilla**
**1 Cup Sourdough Starter**
**1 Cup Unrefined Sugar**
**½ Cup Flour (Whole Wheat or Sorghum)**
**½ Cup Oats**
**½ t Salt**

Melt the butter and whisk in the cocoa. In a large bowl, beat cocoa and butter into the eggs, vanilla, starter, and sugar.

In a separate bowl, whisk together the flour, oats, and salt. Add the flour mix to the wet ingredients and gently fold them in.

Allow to rise for 30 minutes in a warm place.

Bake 17-20 minutes at 350°.

This recipe is also yummy with ½ cup chopped dried cherries, chocolate chips, or peanut butter mixed in after folding the ingredients.

# MARINADE

*This marinade is not only scrumptious, it is packed with enzymes to help tenderize whatever you drench in it.*

**¾ Cup Dregs**
**¼ Cup Olive Oil**
**¼ Cup Herbal Vinegar**
**3 Cloves Pressed Garlic**
**1/2" or so Grated Ginger**
**1 Teaspoon Sugar**
**Salt and Pepper to Taste**

Mix all ingredients and pour over meat or tofu. Refrigerate a few hours or overnight.

# Appendix A

## Roasting Roots and Grains

There are many roots and grains that can be roasted to enhance the flavor of your beers. Dandelion, burdock, chicory, licorice, and grains like quinoa, amaranth, and millet are all good choices.

You can dig up your own roots, wash them, chop them really small, and then roast them according to the directions below. Or, you can buy any of these dried and chopped, and roast them yourself.

One method uses a stovetop popcorn popper, called a Whirley Pop. This is faster and easier than the oven method. Just put whatever you want to roast into the popper, with the stove on low to medium heat. Turn the crank until the contents are the color you want them to be. It's just that easy! I find Whirley Pops at thrift stores all of the time. They also roasts nuts and coffee beans!

The oven method just takes a bit longer, but it is still pretty easy. Spread the roots or grains out on a pan and bake on 250° (with the oven door slightly open if the roots are fresh- to let moisture escape).

Keep an eye on things, and remove when they are the color you want. If you started with fresh roots, this will take about 2 hours. From dry, it will be a lot faster, maybe 20 minutes.

# Appendix B

## Herb and Brewing Resources

# Herb Seeds and Plants

Horizon Herbs, LLC
PO Box 69
Williams, OR 97544 USA
http://www.horizonherbs.com/

RICHTERS HERBS
357 Highway 47
Goodwood, ON L0C 1A0 Canada
Tel. +1.905.640.6677
http://www.richters.com

# Herbs

Pacific Botanicals
4840 Fish Hatchery Road
Grants Pass, OR 97527
Telephone (541) 479-7777
http://www.pacificbotanicals.com


Sunstar Herbs
417 Camino Cerro Chato
Cerillos NM 87010
becky@sunstarherbs.net
*A source for hard to find jujube dates!!*

# Brewing Supplies

Seven Bridges Cooperative
325A River Street
Santa Cruz, CA 95060

http://www.breworganic.com

*The world's only cooperatively owned, certified organic homebrew supply store.*

# Bibliography & Further Reading

## Articles

McGovern, P.E., J. Zhang, J. Tang, Z. Zhang, G. R. Hall, R. A. Moreau, A. Nuñez, E. D. Butrym, M. P. Richards, C.-s. Wang, G. Cheng, Z. Zhao, and C. Wang. "Fermented Beverages of Pre- and Proto-Historic China." Proceedings of the National Academy of Sciences USA 101.51 (2004): 17593-98.

McGovern, P.E., M. Christofidou-Solomidou, W. Wang, F. Dukes, T. Davidson, and W.S. El-Deiry. "Anticancer Activity of Botanical Compounds in Ancient Fermented Beverages." International Journal of Oncology 37(1), ( 2010) 5-21.

McGovern, P.E., R. H. Michel, V. R. Badler. "Chemical Evidence for Ancient Beer." Nature 360 (Nov. 5, 1992): 24.

McGovern, P.E., R. H. Michel, V. R. Badler. "The First Wine and Beer: Chemical Detection of Ancient Fermented Beverages." Analytical Chemistry 65(1993): 408A-413A.

## Books

Buhner, S.H. Sacred and Herbal Healing Beers: The Secrets of Ancient Fermentation. Boulder, CO: Siris. 1993.

Clotfelter, Susan. The Herb Tea Book. Interweave Press. 1998.

Fisher, Joe and Dennis Fisher. The Homebrewer's Garden. Storey Publishing. 1998

Garran, Thomas Avery. Western Herbs According to Traditional Chinese Medicine. Healing Arts Press. 2008.

Gladstar, Rosemary. Rosemary Gladstar's Herbal Recipes for Vibrant Health: 175 Teas, Tonics, Oils, Salves, Tinctures, and Other Natural Remedies for the Entire Family. Storey Publishing. 2008.

Green, James. The Herbal Medicine-Maker's Handbook: A Home Manual. Crossing Press. 2000.

Katz, Sandor Ellix. "Wild Fermentation: The Flavor, Nutrition, and Craft of Live-Culture Foods" Chelsea Green. 2003.

La Pense, Clive. The Historical Companion to Housewbrewing. Beverly, U.K.: Montag Publications. 1990.

McGovern, P.E. Uncorking The Past. University of California Press. 1993.

Papazian, Charlie. The Homebrewer's Companion. New York: Avon Books. 1994.

Tierra, Lesley. Healing With the Herbs of Life. Crossing Press. 2003.

Tierra, Michael. Planetary Herbology. Lotus Press. 1992.

Zak, Victoria. 20,000 Secrets of Tea: The Most Effective Ways to Benefit from Nature's Healing Herbs. Dell. 1999.

# Index

Airlock, 5
All Grain Brewing, 28, 42
Beer
    history, 1
    Recipes, 37-50
    styles, 24-30
Bitters, 11
Bottling, 21-23
Brewing Stages, 18
Brownies!, 55
Brushes, 7, 16, 17
Burdock, 33, 36, 40, 46, 57
Crepes, 54
Dandelion Stout, 46
Dandelions, 11, 33, 40, 45, 46, 57
Dregs, 21, 28, 51-56
Dry Malt Extract, DME, 10
Elderberry Porter, 50
Equipment, 4-8
Extract Brewing, 10, 24-28, 38-41
Extracts, 10
Fermentation, 20-21
Formulating, 31-36
Fruits, 13
Gluten-free, 10, 21, 38, 52, 53
Grains, 9-10
Head Space 23
Herbs, 13
Hops, 11
Hydrometer, 6-7
Ingredients, 9-14
Licorice, 33, 40, 44, 45, 50
Liquid Malt Extract, LME, 10

Malts, 9-10
Marinade, 56
Nettles Spring Ale, 40
Partial Mash, 30, 47-50
Pitching, 19-20
Planetary Porter, 45
Priming, 21, 27
Roman Ale, 49
Sanitizer, 15-17
Second Treasure Tonic, 44
Siphoning, 22-23, 28
Sourdough, 53-55
Stopper, 5-6
Straining Wort, 14
Yeast, 11-12
Yi Sheng's Brew, 41

Made in the USA
San Bernardino, CA
31 August 2014